HOW TO IMPROVE YOUR DIGESTION AND ABSORPTION

Christopher Scarfe

THE **nutrition CONNECTION**

First published in 1989
by ION Press,
a division of The Institute for Optimum Nutrition
5 Jerdan Place, London SW6 1BE

Cover Design : QA

ISBN 1 870976 03 7

Printed and bound in Great Britain by
Brier Press, High Wycombe, Bucks

CONTENTS

IMPROVING DIGESTION   5

Your Digestive System - A Guided Tour   6
Understanding Digestion   9
Digestive Enzymes - Nature's Demolition Team   10
Indigestion - Too Much or Too Little Acid?   12

IMPROVING ABSORPTION   15

Understanding Absorption   16
Your Bacteria in the Balance   17
Candida Albicans - A Beastly Yeast   19
Food Allergies - Your Hidden Enemy   20
Promoting Bowel Regularity   23

EATING TO RESTORE DIGESTIVE HEALTH   27

Raw Energy   27
Food Combining for Health   29
Supplementary Benefits   33

YOUR PERSONAL CLEANSING PROGRAMME   35

Internal Cleansing   35
Maximising Digestion   38
Controlling Candida Albicans   39
Your Thirty Day Spring Clean   43

ABOUT THE AUTHOR

Christopher Scarfe entered the field of nutrition as a response to his wife's rheumatoid arthritis . They wanted to find a safe alternative to the medication being offered, and began to read and experiment with diet and supplementation with very encouraging results. In 1986 he qualified as a nutritionist at ION with 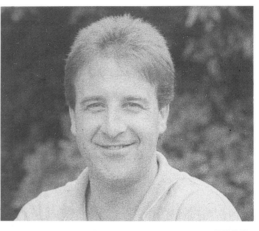 the highest distinction. He started to see clients, soon joining ION's team of consultants, specialising in digestive disorders and arthritis. He also began to teach at the Institute and found a great interest in the importance of the digestive system in human health. In 1987 he was appointed co-director of the Institute for Optimum Nutrition.

Now 35 years old he has contributed to a number of national magazines and teaches both in Britain and abroad. He lives in London with his wife and eight year old daughter and balances his family and working life with a keen interest in the martial arts, in which he is also an experienced teacher.

CHAPTER ONE

IMPROVING DIGESTION

So why do we eat? The simple answer is - in order to provide ourselves with good quality raw materials to sustain life. But there can be a variety of different answers to this question depending on the individual and the circumstances. Because we are hungry, because we crave a certain taste or texture, because we are upset, because it is time to eat, because we see or smell food, because our blood sugar level needs topping up. These are all reasons why we may, at any time, feel the need to eat.

Whatever the reason, for most of us, eating is a fairly unconscious process and the food that we select is often not what our bodies need for nourishment. As a result of this we can end up short of nutrients and risk damage to our digestive systems.

It can be argued that the digestive system is the most important system in our bodies. After all we rely on it to provide us with the raw materials needed for energy, growth, repair and reproduction.

It is robust but has a delicate structure. It is diverse, performing complex feats of demolition with a minimum of effort. It produces 9 litres of digestive fluids every day to lubricate and provide the right environment for the ordered dismantling of nature's energy puzzle. With a better understanding of what your digestive system is and how it works you can learn to support it and encourage it to do the vital work that it is trying to do. When this happens you can benefit from the real nourishment and vitality from food that nature intended.

YOUR DIGESTIVE SYSTEM - A GUIDED TOUR

Your digestive system includes the gastrointestinal tract (GI tract) - *mouth, oesophagus, stomach, small intestine, large intestine* - and the glandular organs - *salivary glands, liver, gallbladder* and *pancreas* which secrete digestive fluids into the GI tract.

The GI tract is a tube approximately 15ft long running through the body. The lumen, rather like the hole inside a hose pipe, is continuous with the external environment - which means that the contents are technically outside the body. This fact is relevant to an understanding of some of the properties of the GI tract. For example, we have billions of bacteria in our colon, accounting for between three and four pounds of our body weight. They are generally beneficial and perform some very important functions but will cause havoc if they gain entry to the body. This might happen, for example, if the appendix gets ruptured - a potentially life threatening situation.

The Mouth

The mouth provides a means for tearing and grinding food. Salivary glands under the tongue and in the top of the cheeks secrete saliva which provides lubrication, enabling the food to pass down the oesophagus and into the stomach.

The Stomach

Now the food is mixed with digestive juices and churned by the muscular walls of the stomach. The resulting *chyme* takes anything from two to five hours to completely leave the stomach. This depends upon the kind of food eaten. At least part of the function of the stomach is to store chyme, while digestive juices do their work.

IMPROVING DIGESTION

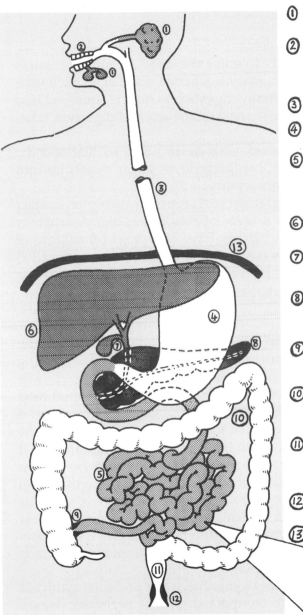

Figure 1 - The Digestive System

① **SALIVARY GLANDS**
SECRETE SALIVARY AMYLASE.

② **TEETH**
INCISORS and CANINES FOR CUTTING:
MOLARS FOR CHEWING.

③ **OESOPHAGUS**

④ **STOMACH**
SECRETES ACID and ENZYMES.

⑤ **SMALL INTESTINE**
SECRETES DIGESTIVE JUICES. SQUEEZES FOOD THROUGH. MOST ABSORPTION OCCURS HERE.

⑥ **LIVER**
PRODUCES BILE.

⑦ **GALLBLADDER**
SECRETES BILE INTO THE SMALL INTESTINE.

⑧ **PANCREAS**
SECRETES DIGESTIVE ENZYMES and SALTS INTO SMALL INTESTINE.

⑨ **ILEO-CAECAL VALVE**
SEPARATES SMALL and LARGE INTESTINE.

⑩ **COLON**
HOME OF FRIENDLY and NOT SO FRIENDLY BACTERIA. OUR WASTE DISPOSAL ORGAN.

⑪ **RECTUM**
WHEN WASTE ARRIVES HERE, DEFAECATION IS STIMULATED.

⑫ **ANUS**
MUSCULAR VALVE

⑬ **DIAPHRAGM**

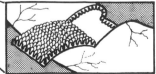

DETAIL OF VILLI IN A CROSS-SECTION OF SMALL INTESTINE

The Small Intestine

The chyme is now ready to enter the small intestine which is composed of three parts - *duodenum, jejunum* and *ileum* , each with different functions. The partially digested mixture is squeezed into the duodenum. This is where most of the work of digestion takes place.

Here the chyme is mixed with more juices so that specific enzymes can do their work, breaking down larger molecules into their component parts for absorption.

In order to provide the greatest surface area possible for contact with the gut wall, there is a layer of tiny finger-like protrusions called *villi* which line the small intestine. This provides millions of enzyme secreting cells. It is estimated to give a surface area of 300 square metres, (equivalent to the area of a tennis court), for the absorption of nutrients.

The Colon

The food is moved from one end of the small intestine to the other by waves of muscular contractions called *peristalsis* ; during this time most of the nourishment is absorbed from the food. The remaining material, including undigested fibres, unabsorbed food components and dead cells, arrives at the junction of the small and large intestines (the *ileum* and *caecum*) - the *ileo caecal valve*. The correct functioning of this valve is of particular importance as it allows the passage of chyme into the large intestine, or *colon* , whilst preventing the passage of faeces and bacteria back into the small intestine. Many factors about our modern lifestyle and eating habits can interfere with the function of this valve, resulting in a back flow of faecal material into the small intestine. This can give rise to auto-intoxication (self poisoning) and unpleasant symptoms. More is said about this in the next chapter.

On reaching the colon, the chyme has water and salts extracted from it and becomes more compacted. Strong peristaltic waves move the faecal matter along the colon for defaecation. As the colon stores waste matter it is exposed to a higher concentration of toxic material than other parts of the digestive tract. This is particularly relevant when there is constipation, as this increases the risk of diseases of the colon.

The time taken for food to pass from mouth to anus should be twelve to twenty four hours. The reflex to defaecate is stimulated by the presence of faeces in the rectum and also by the entry of food into the stomach. It is important for optimum health that this reflex is not consciously over-ridden as this can result in inhibition of defaecation, resulting in constipation. This is particularly important for children as they can learn to become constipated adults.

UNDERSTANDING DIGESTION

The Russian researcher Pavlov was able to cause dogs to salivate with the stimulus of a bell by first teaching them that the sound of the bell heralded dinner. He would then ring the bell and provide no dinner but the dogs would still salivate. The same is true of us, subtle stimuli, like the thought of a tasty meal, are at work causing the secretion of digestive juices before we even take our first bite. Being prepared for a meal and thinking good thoughts about it can be important factors in the subsequent quality of the digestive process.

We consume most of our food as large particles such as proteins, carbohydrates and fats, but our metabolism requires the presence of smaller particles such as amino acids, sugars and fatty acids in order to perform the myriad of functions that we call life. The stepwise dismantling of these large particles is achieved by the presence of digestive enzymes (nature's demolition team) and the accompanying correct acidic or alkaline environment.

The GI tract has evolved to maximise the absorption of the substances in our food and generally will attempt to digest and absorb everything that is put into it.

Its efficiency depends on the type of foods eaten, the quantity of digestive enzymes secreted, the presence or absence of certain digestive inhibitory factors, muscular health for proper peristalsis and the correct acid/alkaline environment for enzymes.

For example, in nature, carbohydrates (long chains of sugars or starches) appear in the complex form, that is in a matrix of indigestible materials which we call fibre. This promotes digestive health by providing bulk for the digestive muscles to work on. It also provides a carrier for the removal of dead cells and mucus, and makes it relatively hard for the enzymes to get at the digestible carbohydrates thus providing for the slow release of sugars into the bloodstream. Complex carbohydrate foods also provide the co-factors required for the digestion, absorption and subsequent metabolism of the sugars released, namely vitamins and minerals.

If we refine carbohydrates and remove the fibre we are left with a concentrated source of sugar which is too easy for enzymes to digest. Refined carbohydrates include white flour and its products, white rice and sugar. These processed foods give an inappropriate fast release of sugars into the blood and a fibre-less sludge which is hard for the muscles of the intestine to remove. This sludge can easily fill up the tiny spaces between the villi, inhibiting digestion and absorption. Processed foods also fail to provide adequate levels of the vitamins and minerals that our bodies need for making more digestive enzymes and for turning glucose into energy. This sets up a vicious cycle of declining digestive efficiency.

Understanding that factors, such as stress and low stomach acid, exist and that their reduction improves digestion, is fundamental for improving the absorption of the goodness in our food.

DIGESTIVE ENZYMES - NATURE'S DEMOLITION TEAM

Think of fats, proteins and carbohydrates as long chains of different coloured balls (molecules) connected with string (bonds). Between any two given balls the string may be of a different thickness. To break these chains up we need pairs of scissors of different gauges. This is what digestive enzymes do. The different parts of the GI tract provide different types of chemical scissors.

In The Mouth

Very little digestion occurs here as there is only a weak *amylase*

(-ase denotes an enzyme), or starch splitting enzyme, present and the time that food spends in the mouth does not give salivary amylase much chance to work. Little importance is ever placed on the proper chewing of food, though we would enjoy our food more, and allow more time for the secretion of other digestive juices, if we did pay attention to chewing, which also enhances our sense of taste.

In The Stomach

This is where protein digestion begins. Cells lining the walls of the stomach secrete a strong acid, *hydrochloric acid*, which unravels the tightly wound spiral chains in which protein normally appears. Once this has occurred then a *protease* (protein splitting enzyme) called *pepsin* , is better able to get access to the chains of amino acids making up the protein. It then chops these very long chains of amino acids into smaller chains called *polypeptides* .

In infants, *rennin* is present which clots milk, rendering it more easily digested - though its presence diminishes as the infant grows up and is weaned onto solid foods. If milk continues to be part of the diet then this encourages the production of rennin into adulthood. Milk allergy is connected with poor digestion and may result from a lack of rennin.

Little carbohydrate digestion takes place in the stomach as the acid tends to neutralise salivary amylase.

In The Duodenum

The chyme which is squirted into the duodenum is highly acidic and needs to be altered, as the enzymes of the small intestine will only work in an alkaline medium. In order to bring this about there are three sources of secretions.

The liver manufactures bile, which contains alkaline salts, and is stored and concentrated in the gall bladder. The pancreas and the walls of the duodenum also secrete alkaline salts which, together with the concentrated bile from the gall bladder, neutralise the acid chyme from the stomach and provide an alkaline environment. One of the most important properties of bile is its ability to emulsify large dietary fat globules into much smaller fat droplets, so that lipase can go to work dismantling the individual fat molecules. Here in the duodenum all starches will be broken down to single sugar molecules (*monosaccharides*) by the action of amylases ready for absorption. Most of this is the monosaccharide glucose. Some will be fructose from fruits and vegetables.

Polypeptides, resulting from protein digestion in the stomach, are also broken down here, by the action of protease and peptidase enzymes.

These three fundamental groups of enzymes secreted by the pancreas and duodenal cells are shown in Figure 2.

INDIGESTION - TOO MUCH OR TOO LITTLE ACID?

Indigestion is the term most often used to describe discomfort in the digestive system. It is a non-specific term and usually refers to problems in the stomach. Most commonly it is   assumed that this arises out of an excess of hydrocholoric acid in the stomach. The remedy is usually antacid medication containing alkaline salts which help to reduce the assumed excess acidity in the stomach. There is usually some reduction in sypmtoms such as pain, wind, bloating and heartburn.

Though excess stomach acidity does occur, and may be the cause of gastric ulcers, it is much more common for indigestion to be the result of low levels of stomach acid.

If acid secretion is inadequate, food can remain in the stomach for longer than it should and the carbohydrate can begin to ferment and produce gas. Bad breath and belching can be indicators of this condition. In this case, it is more appropriate to provide hydrochloric acid supplements. This would encourage the proper digestion of food and the consequent absorption of adequate zinc and B6, both needed for the production of good levels of stomach acid.

Ironically, antacid preparations, can provide relief for people with a lack of stomach acid. The mechanism is quite simple. If stomach acid levels are already low and you introduce large amounts

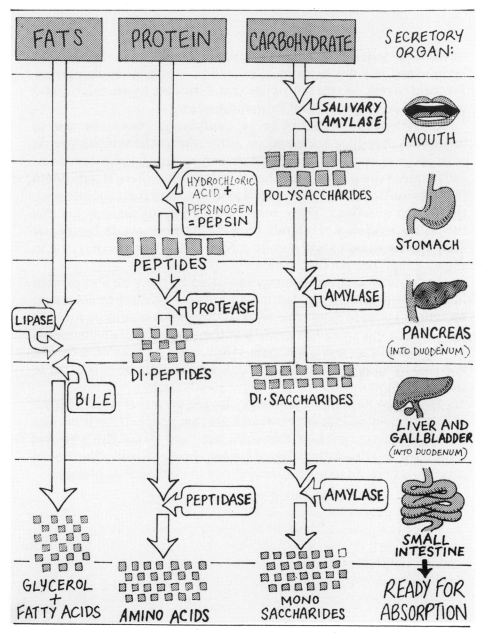

Figure 2 - The Action of Digestive Enzymes

13

of alkaline salts, the acid level will drop even further. Now the body's feedback mechanisms come into play and, recognising very low acid levels, secrete hormones that stimulate hydrochloric acid release. Thus there is relief from indigestion.

It is therefore wise not to be complacent about the use of antacids. Often they are based on aluminium salts which provide toxic levels of aluminium if used frequently. Also, if there is the need for frequent use of such aids then it follows that there is a problem in the manufacture of hydrochloric acid - too much or too little acid, that is the question. There may be a variety of reasons for this including deficiency of vitamin B6 and zinc, hormone imbalance or simple exhaustion of acid secreting cells after a lifetime of trying to digest a high protein diet.

Excess stomach acid can be stimulated by diets high in protein or excess production of histamine, a hormone which stimulates acid secretion. If excess stomach acid is discovered it would be more to the point to reduce excess protein in the diet or balance histamine levels rather than using antacids. High levels of histamine can be reduced by adding calcium, vitamin C and vitamin B6 to the diet in moderate amounts.

Many people hold the seemingly logical view that liquids drunk with a meal will dilute enzymes and prevent proper digestion. The evidence is clear, however, that sufficient fluid taken with a meal is important in stimulating digestive responses. Ideally the liquid should be at room temperature and not more than two glasses.

CHAPTER TWO

IMPROVING ABSORPTION

Nutrient absorption is not a passive process like a sponge soaking up water. It is a highly specific and energetic activity more akin to the organisation involved when the famous wealthy American bought what he thought was London's Tower Bridge, dismantled it and shipped it to the USA. Like the different components in the bridge, the components of our food have special transport methods by which they gain access to the bloodstream. Also, like the American, we can make the wrong choice of raw materials - he actually bought the old London Bridge.

Good absorption relies on the right conditions prevailing, particularly the cleanliness and health of the tiny villi lining the gut wall. Generally speaking, fat, protein and carbohydrate absorption will proceed even in the most hostile environment. It is the vitamins and minerals that are the most vulnerable to adverse conditions - and we need to absorb them well, as their concentration in our food is ever decreasing.

Many vitamins and minerals are employed as co-workers in this process and are often found in foods which they help to absorb. This is one reason why fresh, and whole food is important.

UNDERSTANDING ABSORPTION

When you consider that many nutrients have a low rate of absorption even under the best conditions, it is easy to see how we might become undernourished on a typical Western diet. With a healthy GI tract it is possible to absorb about 30% of the zinc in food. The average diet in the UK only provides borderline levels of zinc. Couple this with poor absorption and the risk of zinc deficiency is considerable. Zinc has so far been shown to be essential for two hundred different processes in the body including eyesight, sexual potency and protection from cancer. Improving the quality of the food you eat not only helps provide vitamins and minerals, but also helps to create the right conditions for efficient absorption. This may not just promote your health but may save you money too.

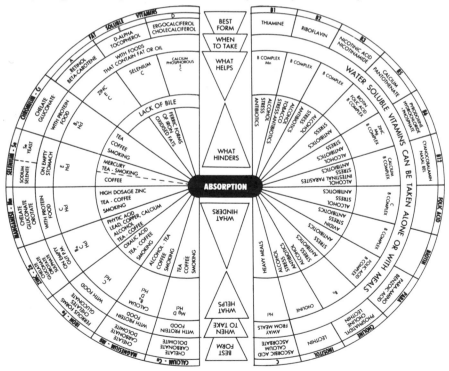

Figure 3 - Maximising Absorption

Tens of millions of pounds are spent on vitamin and mineral supplements every year in the UK. It is estimated that as much as sixty percent of these nutrients are flushed away, excreted as waste because they have not been absorbed. If they are taken under the right conditions, vitamin, mineral and other nutrient supplements can be well absorbed and a worthwhile addition to a healthy diet.

A Veritable Assault Course

The type of food that we eat and the liquids we drink also have a bearing on absorption. Wheat bran binds with calcium and zinc inhibiting their absorption - one reason not to add wheat bran to your diet. Tea and coffee reduce the availability of minerals like calcium, magnesium, zinc and iron. Alcohol interferes with magnesium, zinc and most B vitamins.

Many other environmental factors like tobacco smoke, stress, antibiotics, cooking and pollution (lead directly blocks calcium and zinc absorption), all interefere with the absorption of nutrients. The sludge produced by refined carbohydrates clogs up the tiny spaces between the villi and severely reduces the absorption surface area. All in all, it is a wonder that any nutrients get through this assault course. The good news is that if we apply what we now know about digestion, we can greatly improve the nourishment that we get from our food and run a serious risk of enhancing our health. Conscious eating need not be a labour, it is a tasty and enjoyable way of staying fit and disease free into old age.

YOUR BACTERIA IN THE BALANCE

We are able to live on this planet only by establishing a relationship between the millions of bacteria that live on us and in us. By far the most important concentration of bacteria is in the colon. They perform a wide variety of different functions, including providing immunity, helping detoxification and making some vitamins.

The colon can be considered the waste disposal system of the body. We are constantly pouring potentially toxic waste products of digestion into it, and if we fail to empty this regularly the consequence will be overflow. In our colon this takes the form of faecal backflow into the small intestine as well as reabsorption of toxins through the wall of the colon. In order for this waste to be properly dealt with the intestinal bacteria, must be in the correct balance.

There are two different types of bacteria that inhabit the colon. They are the bifido strain, which are essentially beneficial, and the bacteroides strain, which are responsible for putrefaction (decomposing food particles that reach the colon). The balance should be about 85% to 15% in favour of the beneficial strains.

Many aspects of our modern lifestyle cause a disruption of this balance in favour of the putrefactive strains which produce gases and toxic wastes themselves. Excess flatulence is the first sign that this is happening. Once wastes re-enter the bloodstream they can cause a variety of symptoms such as fatigue, poor concentration, irritability, insomnia, headaches, muscle aches, joint pain and stiffness, and often contribute to the onset of degenerative diseases. Here are some of the factors that favour an increase in the putrefactive bacteria:

- Antibiotics (both from medication and residues in meat)
- High fat and protein diets (especially meat, fish and eggs)
- Stress
- Sugar consumption
- Lack of dietary fibre
- Excess alcohol consumption
- Lack of exercise
- Stimulants such as tea and coffee
- Diets high in processed foods and dairy products.

Antibiotics appear to present the biggest problem; as although they are effective in killing alien bacteria, they also do a good job of killing off large numbers of our beneficial gut bacteria.

Breast is Best

It has been shown that babies that are breast fed have a much better bacterial balance than babies that are fed on cows milk. Breast fed babies have a better chance of becoming healthy adults as their digestive systems will work more efficiently - that is if they do not destroy their bacteria by the negative factors above. Breast feeding is the most important factor in the subsequent intestinal health of the individual.

The second most important factor is diet. Indigestible fibre from vegetables, pulses, nuts, seeds, grains and fruits provides bulk that encourages the correct transit time for faeces. When the passage of faeces slows down we get constipated - from the Latin word for compacting or cramming. Most researchers in this field agree that most Western folk are constipated, since basic rural populations (such as those still found in Africa) who live on simple food, will have two or three bowel movements daily. The incidence of Western type degenerative diseases such as cancer and arthritis are almost unheard of there, except in places exposed to Western diets.

So, by keeping your bacteria balanced, you prevent the colonisation of disease causing micro-ogranisms, limit the toxic waste products of the putrefactive bacteria and stimulate proper peristalsis for the expulsion of faeces.

Once the bacterial balance has been disrupted the way is laid open for opportunistic micro-organisms to take advantage of the warm moist and nutritious environment prevailing in your colon.

CANDIDA ALBICANS - A BEASTLY YEAST

The common yeast, Candida Albicans, is one such micro-organism. This yeast is to be found everywhere in nature and is found in the intestinal flora of healthy humans, but in very small quantities. Only one purpose has so far been found for this yeast. When we die it initiates the process of decomposition. However if conditions in the intestines become favourable for it while we are alive then it will begin to decompose our intestinal contents and us before our time.

When the right conditions prevail, Candida Albicans changes from its yeast form into its fungal form, whereupon it sends out tiny roots that penetrate the cells of the gut wall, damaging them and causing the gut wall to become permeable to chemicals and other micro-organisms that it would normally provide protection against. Fermentation and the production of toxic waste products cause gases and create the wrong environment for our beneficial bacteria, so their numbers fall. Eventually we have a reduced ability to fight off any invading organisms. Having lost our first line of defence the internal immune system now has to deal with an increasing number of dangerous aliens. Now we become prone to common, but normally combated, viruses, because our immune system is busy dealing with other aliens in our bloodstream.

The consequences of Candida Albicans infestation, called *candidiasis*, are far reaching and can account for a wide variety of symptoms. Candida Albicans can also migrate into the blood and be carried to all other parts of the body, it may then thrive in other body tissues and interfere with their proper function.

Like the putrefactive bacteria, Candida Albicans loves a diet high in refined carbohydrates, sugar, alcohol, tea, coffee and dairy products, along with a stressful and polluted lifestyle.

FOOD ALLERGIES - YOUR HIDDEN ENEMY

The purpose of our immune system is to recognise anything alien in the body and neutralise it. Rather like a conventional modern army it has specialised units for blocking the alien's access or dealing with it once it has breached the first lines of defence. The common allergic reaction, hay fever, demonstrates this well. Pollen, the *allergen* (a substances that provokes an allergic response) from grass or trees, enters the lungs. Firstly, we sneeze to try to expel the irritant. If this is unsuccessful the next symptoms to appear are itching eyes, sore throat, runny nose and blocked sinuses, from the inflammatory effects of histamine (you will note that these symptoms are identical with those of the common cold, and often people with frequent reactions like these, outside the hay fever season, believe they are getting frequent colds and flu when they are actually suffering food allergy reactions). Often, anti-histamine drugs are given to relieve these symptoms. Once inside the blood, the allergen may provoke much stronger symptoms such as anxiety,

Could Yeast Be Your Problem?

If you have a health problem that you suspect may be associated with Candida Albicans then see how you score on the following questionnaire:

- Do you have a history of frequent courses of antibiotics?
- Have you had prolonged exposure to steroid medication or the birth control pill?
- Do you crave sweet things, bread or alcoholic beverages?
- Are you subject to frequent minor infections?
- Do you have allergies?
- Do you have a history of thrush, anal itch or athletes foot?
- Do you suffer from premenstrual syndrome (PMS), loss of libido, prostitis, vaginitis or cystitis?
- Have you learned to live with fatigue, depression, poor memory, confusion or nerves?
- Do you have muscle aches, joint pain, numb patches, headaches or blurred vision?

If you answer yes to 5 or 6 of these questions then your health problem is probably due to yeasts.

If you answer yes to 7 or more then your symptoms are almost definitely due to yeasts.

Many medical authorities are sceptical about the connection of yeasts with a wide variety of disorders, ranging from irritable bowel syndrome to schizophrenia, but the evidence is very strong in favour of such a connection.

confusion, headache, lack of energy and even depression.

Similarly, under the right conditions, it is possible for components of our food, or chemicals, to enter the blood from the digestive system and provoke an immune response. Apart from the extreme reactions that some people have to strawberries, lobster and other specific foods, there is a far more common reaction to hidden food allergens that appear daily in the diet and are often not recognised as causing problems.

The following factors increase the potential for food allergy or intolerance:
- Vitamin, mineral and essential fatty acid deficiency
- Low fibre diets
- Low stomach acid production
- Poor pancreatic enzyme production
- Long term drug medication
- Stress
- Pollution
- Addiction
- Imbalance of intestinal bacteria
- Candida Albicans infestation

More than 2,000 years ago the Roman physician Lucretius commented "what may be food to one may be fierce poison to others". Then, this was probably a rare observation, but today, with increasing reports of food allergy, or intolerance, medical science is beginning to recognise our individuality and potential for altered responses to common foods.

Symptoms associated with food allergy include hyperactivity (especially in children), mood swings, anxiety, depression, poor concentration, headaches, joint and muscle aches, irritable bowel syndrome, insomnia, eczema, asthma, palpitations and lethargy. There are many, many more.

A wide variety of therapeutic approaches, not the least important of which is nutrition, can help in the treatment of food allergy. Many of the other ways of dealing with allergies, however, only deal with the symptoms and not with the root cause.

In Defence of Your Realm

To prevent or treat allergies it is vital to strengthen the immune system's first lines of defence, so that food particles cannot gain access to the blood. It is most commonly improperly digested protein particles, called peptides, that gain entry to the blood and cause allergic symptoms.

Prevention may be supported by eating wholefoods, reducing

stress and avoidable stressors like sugar, caffeine and nicotine, and by eating a wide variety of foods rather than accepting a diet that is based on a few major ingredients, such as wheat, dairy products, sugar and saturated fats.

The treatment of food allergies will nearly always also require temporary removal of the allergen from the diet, in order to give the digestive and immune system the opportunity to recover and become balanced. Changes to diet and supplementation can then help to strengthen the body and replenish nutrient deficiencies.

So how do you isolate the foods that might be causing you a problem? Unfortunately it is usually the foods that we most like and would find hardest to give up that are the culprits. Also, foods that are most commonly eaten and that are used as components of other prepared foods should be suspected. The most common food allergens in the UK are: wheat and its products, dairy products, eggs, sugar, chocolate, citrus fruits and food colouring - this is at least partly due to the fact that these foods are frequently eaten. In the USA, where corn and its flour is more often eaten than wheat, corn is at the top of the list.

You will know if a suspected food is an allergen if you feel better once it has been removed from your diet. Often people resist finding out what their food allergies are because they fear that they will then never be able to eat their favourite foods again. This is not so, as most allergic sufferers are able to tolerate their allergen in moderation once they have improved their digestion and absorption, strengthened their immune systems, replenished nutrient deficiencies and adjusted to a more wholesome and natural diet and lifestyle.

PROMOTING BOWEL REGULARITY

Dr Dennis Burkitt is the man responsible for putting dietary fibre on the map. He spent quite some time in the late 1950's assessing the stool quality of various African rural communities and comparing them with stool samples from Westerners hospitalised with a variety of disorders, ranging from diabetes to haemorrhoids.

What he found was that African communities, living on a

The Pulse Test

Here is a very simple test that you can use to assess a food allergy. Avoid the suspected food for at least 14 days - this must be done rigorously by being aware of the foods that contain your suspected allergen. This means reading labels and stocking up on substitutes so that you do not get caught out. Then put aside an hour or so and sit in a comfortable chair with a watch, pencil and paper and a good dose of your allergen. For example a large glass of milk or a doorstep of your favourite bread would suffice.

Record your resting pulse after 15 minutes seated. Now eat your allergen. Record your pulse again at ten, thirty and sixty minute intervals. You must remain seated throughout. Do not smoke or consume anything else during this time.

Over the next forty eight hours you should record any unusual symptoms. The combination of a change of ten or more beats in your pulse, up or down, with the appearance of symptoms would be convincing evidence in support of food allergy. If you do get such a positive response you should avoid that food and follow the recommendations in chapter four. If you suspect other allergies then this procedure can be repeated for each food. After six months or so, you should be able to reintroduce the food back into your diet, being careful not to eat it every day , as this may take you back to square one.

traditional diet, occasionally supplemented with a little meat, fish or dairy produce, produced soft, bulky and fibrous stools, two or three times daily. The prevalence of Western type diseases, such as heart disease, cancer, diabetes and disorders of the bowels, were in the order of fractions of one percent of the population.

The hospitalised Westerners, on the other hand, had a diet of refined carbohydrates, sugar, saturated fat, meat, dairy products and salt. Here he found stools that were hard, compacted and dense and passed at best once a day (often with difficulty) and sometimes as little as once a week.

Apart from contributing to our major killer degenerative diseases, irregular bowel function has since been established as a major factor in the cause of disorders of the bowel such as: constipation, diarrhoea, haemorrhoids, irritable bowel syndrome, colitis, diverticulitis, Crohn's disease and cancer of the large bowel.

How then, in the context of our modern way of life, can we seek to promote bowel regularity and prevent and help to treat, common Western diseases?

Dr Burkitt, and those who have been inspired by him to study other non-Westernised communities, suggest that we can learn much from the more primitive lifestyle and natural eating habits practised by these human groups.

Though there are dozens of factors affecting bowel regularity the fundamental ones are described below.

Fibrous Foods

Firstly, it is clear that we can change our refined and animal produce oriented diet for one that is composed of highly fibrous vegetables, roots, grains, pulses, seeds and fruits. This single factor on its own also promotes digestive juices and better absorption. It also provides the right environment for our beneficial bacteria, and we have seen how important these are. There is no substitute for unrefined, natural and vital foods!

The Importance of Exercise

When we inhale, the diaphragm (a flat muscle separating the chest from the belly) pushes down on the intestines and massages them. When we exhale, we pull our stomach muscles in, pushing waste air out of the lungs and again massaging the intestines. This stimulates the passage of food and faeces, encouraging decreased transit time and reducing the potential for toxic reactions from faeces trapped in the colon.

Most adults do not breathe like this, but have learned to breathe by expanding the chest. Aerobic (oxygen using) exercise encourages the proper use of the diaphragm, aiding digestion. In this way the physical movement associated with brisk walking, running, cycling, swimming and dancing helps promote proper bowel function. Three twenty minute sessions a week is a good basic level.

No Need For Meat

It is clear that our dentition is that of an omnivore (meat and plant eater). However our GI tract is much more like that of a herbivore than a carnivore. The big cats, for example, have a GI tract one third the length of ours. This allows for speedy explusion of waste resulting from animal protein and fat. Our GI tract is only able to cope with small, infrequent amounts of animal produce. The sudden change in our diet towards one high in meat, fish and dairy produce and low in plant foods tends towards low fibre and high fat. This slows transit time, increases putrifactive bacteria and promotes disease in the GI tract. We also eat all of our meat cooked, which reduces the vitamins and minerals available for absorption.

Beneficial Bacteria

Early in this century it was recognised that Bulgarians consuming live yoghurt regularly were very healthy. It was then realised that the reason for this was the assistance offered by the bacteria in their milk cultures in helping beneficial bacteria to thrive in their colons. These lactobaccilli (bacteria cultured in milk) do not take up residence in the colon but are transient, offering temporary assistance if consumed on a regular basis. The use of milk cultures like kefir and yoghurt has also been shown to be effective in diminishing Candida Albicans infestation. Supplements of concentrated cultures of these types of transient bacteria have been available for some years and have proved very useful in the promotion of bowel health, and the prevention and treatment of maldigestion, malabsorption, constipation, diarrhoea, flatulence and allergies.

Recently Swedish researchers have been able to develop human bacterial strains in the laboratory. These are not transient but take up residence in the gut adding to the colonies of beneficial bacteria, increasing the overall health of the digestive system in the long term. These are now commercially available and may prove to be a major factor in the promotion of optimum bowel health in Western society.

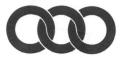

CHAPTER THREE

EATING TO RESTORE DIGESTIVE HEALTH

Y ou are not what you eat. You are what you can digest and absorb. History shows us that we have evolved from raw-plant eating primates to our present civilised state over 30 million years. It should be no surprise that this "primitive" diet is the easiest for us to digest and absorb. Only relatively recently have we learned to cook meats and refine food for making tasty cooked combinations. There is no guarantee that we have evolved the digestive mechanisms to deal with cooked food well - in fact the evidence is to the contrary. We are the only creatures on this planet to display such behaviour and it may be doing us more harm than we realise.

RAW ENERGY

In the mid 1930's, researchers in Europe demonstrated that young animals fed on refined, cooked foods grew and showed no evidence of disease. However, when these animals reached adulthood, they showed signs of degeneration similar to those demonstrated by humans in Western societies: tooth decay, constipation, large numbers of harmful bacteria in the colon and calcium loss from the bones.

This state was referred to as "meso-health", a kind of half-health resulting from years of eating refined and devitalised foods. Once these animals were put onto a diet containing plenty of fresh green vegetables and cereals their health was very much restored. These researchers recommended that a vast majority of people suffering from degenerative diseases could improve their health by following a similar diet. They also inferred that such a diet would prevent disease.

Many thousands of people have reported improvements in digestive health, energy levels, mental clarity and emotional balance with a diet high in raw, unprocessed and vital foods.

Cooking Can Damage Your Health

Most processed foods have already been cooked and the raw foods that we buy are usually destined for the pot. Many vital nutrients and enzymes present in raw foods are destroyed by cooking. To understand why this may be so, it is important to know a little of what happens to food when it is cooked.

If you heat foods, their complex molecules vibrate until their bonds break and they lose much of their structure. Vitamins often break down and minerals can form salts that we cannot digest. When the bonds of polyunsaturated fat molecules break they can produce toxic forms of oxygen, (free radicals) that promote ageing and cancer. Fibres in carboyhydrate foods lose much of their structure and their starches break down into more simple sugars.

To add insult to injury some of the last vestiges of essential nutrients can be sucked out of our food by frying in fat, boiling in water and charcoal grilling over barbeques. The result is that what we end up eating is very far removed from the life giving, wholesome food from which it was originally prepared. Free radicals (toxic forms of oxygen) are produced if food is overcooked or burnt. The first tissues that they come across are our digestive tissues where there is a real risk of damage. This is a potential cause for the increased incidence of cancer of the colon.

Vitality Foods

When vegetables, fruits, nuts, seeds and sprouts of seeds and pulses are eaten raw they still contain their own enzymes which can aid digestion, taxing our systems less in the process. Nutrients are then provided in their natural context, in good quantities, and without having been denatured by heat and boiling water. Their high fibre content promotes peristalsis and speedy transit time, and encourages a clean GI tract. It takes a lot of nutrients and energy to make the enzymes that are needed for digestion and absorption, so any help we can get from raw foods is good news, and their inclusion in the diet is an important part of promoting digestive health and overall energy levels.

FOOD COMBINING FOR HEALTH

There are more than twenty basic amino acids from which proteins are formed in nature. The human body can manufacture many of these, but must be provided with eight from the diet. These are known as the essential amino acids. With these we can replace old cells, make new ones and make the hormones and enzymes necessary for cell regulation, provided, of course, that we also have an adequate supply of vitamins and minerals to act as co-factors in these metabolic events.

Complementary Proteins

It is therefore important to ensure that the protein portion of the diet provides these eight amino acids. This is not difficult to achieve for most people as meat, fish and dairy produce are sources of complete protein - that is they contain adequate levels of all eight. Vegetable protein, on the other hand, is generally incomplete, not providing all eight amino acids in the right proportions.

Vegetarians, and particularly vegans (who eat no animal products at all), need to select foods that will provide adequate levels of all eight essential amino acids in the course of a day for optimum health. Generally these provisions will be met if foods are selected from a variety of green and yellow vegetables, root vegetables, whole grains, seeds, nuts, sprouted legumes (pulses and beans) and fruits.

Many people who give up meat on spiritual and moral grounds are not aware of this aspect of nutrition and risk deficiency of one or more of the amino acids. The address of the Vegetarian Society is on page 47 for those who require further information on the special aspects of vegetarian diets.

For those of us who eat a variety of foods of animal and vegetable origin it is more important to pay attention to excesses of protein and fat, the wholeness of carbohydrate foods in the diet, and the part they play in digestion and absorption.

The Hay System

Dr William Hay, a country doctor in the USA at the turn of the century, believed that the eating of whole and natural foods was of prime importance in human health. He was given the opportunity to prove this when he became very ill himself and was told by his colleagues that there was no help that they could offer him. He decided to treat himself by "eating fundamentally", eating only those things that he believed nature had intended him to eat, and taking them only in their natural form. To the surprise of his doctors his symptoms gradually went away, he lost weight and felt fitter than he had for many years, all in the space of three months.

Dr Hay went on to practice and refine his ideas with his patients, based on his understanding that no matter how severe or diverse the symptoms of disease, there was only one underlying cause - wrong chemical conditions in the body. These conditions, he said, were created by the accumulation of acidic end-products of metabolism in quantities greater than the body could eliminate.

Acid/Alkaline Balance

All foods provide a residue, or ash, once they have been burned in the body, which is either acid or alkaline. The body is used to dealing with large quantities of alkaline ash and a little acid ash. The foods that provide an alkaline ash are in the main the vegetable foods while meat, fish, dairy products, refined foods and sugar burn to leave an acid ash. This gives us the principle of acid/alkaline balance, a diet composed of 80% alkaline forming and 20% acid forming foods being ideal. Any departure from this balance, Dr Hay believed, would result in acidosis of the blood and a build up of toxins in the tissues. He recognised that many individuals were able to build up a tolerance to this imbalance but did so at considerable cost to their vitality.

Dr Hay advised against mixing starches with proteins or acid fruits at the same meal. Concentrated protein foods (20% or more protein) require an acid medium for digestion (acid fruits provide acid in themselves), and concentrated starches (20% or more starch) require an alkaline medium for digestion. If foods from these two essentially different classes are eaten at the same meal, then the digestive medium has to be wrong for one of them - with the result that one will not be properly digested.

Fundamental Eating

In order to harmonise with the delicate mechanisms of our digestive processes, Dr Hay laid down the following framework:

1. Vegetables, salads and fruits should form the major part of the diet.
2. Only whole grain and unrefined starches should be eaten - all refined foods are taboo, particularly sugar and highly processed fats or margarines.
3. Animal proteins, starches and fats should be eaten in small quantities. Nuts, mushrooms, seeds, yoghurt and sprouted legumes are good sources of protein and can be combined with any foods.
4. Starches (cooked grains and their products, potatoes and sugars) should not be eaten at the same meal as acid fruits or animal proteins.
5. At least four hours should lapse between meals of a different character.

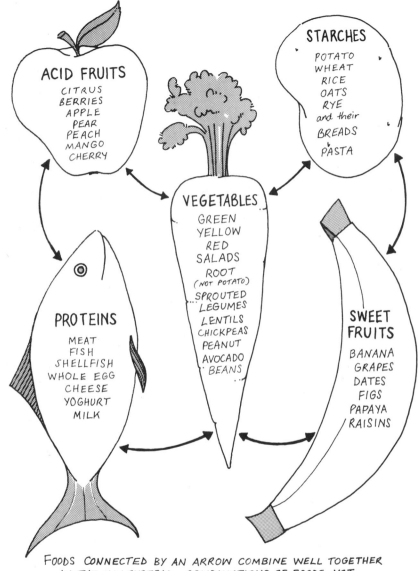

ACID FRUITS
CITRUS
BERRIES
APPLE
PEAR
PEACH
MANGO
CHERRY

STARCHES
POTATO
WHEAT
RICE
OATS
RYE
and their
BREADS
PASTA

VEGETABLES
GREEN
YELLOW
RED
SALADS
ROOT
(NOT POTATO)
SPROUTED
LEGUMES
LENTILS
CHICKPEAS
PEANUT
AVOCADO
BEANS

PROTEINS
MEAT
FISH
SHELLFISH
WHOLE EGG
CHEESE
YOGHURT
MILK

SWEET FRUITS
BANANA
GRAPES
DATES
FIGS
PAPAYA
RAISINS

FOODS CONNECTED BY AN ARROW COMBINE WELL TOGETHER
IN THE HAY SYSTEM. COMBINATIONS OF FOODS NOT
CONNECTED SHOULD BE AVOIDED.

NUTS, SEEDS and MUSHROOMS COMBINE WELL WITH ALL FOODS
AND ARE GOOD SOURCES OF PROTEIN FOR VEGETARIANS.

Figure 4 - Food Combinations - Do's and Don'ts.

Do You Chew or Don't Chew?

As starch digestion is initiated in the mouth, all starch foods must be well chewed in order to mix them with the salivary enzymes. What little protein is in the starch foods is then quickly digested in the stomach and the starchy portion is passed on to the small intestine for digestion. Conversely, when concentrated protein is eaten lots of acid is secreted and the presence of starchy foods will inhibit the action of the acid. Fermentation may then occur in the stomach leading to gas and indigestion. When protein digestion is disrupted, peptides can be absorbed and provoke allergic responses.

Undigested starches reaching the colon are ideal for putrefactive bacteria - the sort that we do not want to encourage. Minor symptoms of an intolerance to mixed foods are flatulence, bloating, lack of energy, bad breath and acid indigestion. Later we may go on to experience allergies, joint aches and pains, headaches, depression, anxiety or any of the hundreds of symptoms so far established as connected with vitamin, and particularly mineral, deficiency.

Eating according to the Hay system automatically promotes acid/alkaline balance, and it is in this chemical balance that Dr Hay and his followers believe lies the secret of real health and resistance to disease. It is also the type of diet we have evolved to consume and one that places the least stress on our digestive processes and enhances absorption. There is recent evidence to support Dr Hay's observation that weight loss is enhanced by eating this way.

SUPPLEMENTARY BENEFITS

"You get all the nourishment you need from a well balanced diet" is another popular misconception. The inference here is that if you select a variety of foods from those offered by the food industry you will be well nourished.

Evidence suggests that peasant diets, even up to the turn of this century, did provide good nourishment alongside low incidence of degenerative, Western type disease. But the way that we grow and present food today is very different. Since the industrial revolution the demand for food has grown in advance of the ability of farmers to supply it. This has generated our current intensive farming and food manufacturing technology, which has led to us eating foods that are deficient in essential vitamins, minerals and fibre. The type of fat that we eat has changed from predominantly unsaturated to predominantly saturated. Crop spray residues, and other air borne toxins like lead and industrial emissions, now contaminate our food too.

Our Changing Needs in a New Environment

The level of stress that we are exposed to from car exhaust fumes, noise, lack of exercise, stimulants like tobacco and alcohol, medical drugs (especially antibiotics), polluted water, hormone residues in meat and dairy produce, toxic metals like lead and aluminium, and the hundreds of other factors that affect our every day lives, places a huge demand on our resources and interferes with our digestive processes.

It is logical then to assume that our needs would differ from those of our ancestors. The fact is that, as stress and pollution have increased, so food quality has diminished. At the same time we have seen an epidemic rise in the incidence of life threatening and degenerative diseases, like cancer (particularly of the bowel), heart disease and arthritis. This is in spite of the achievements claimed by modern medical technology and is especially sad in view of the fact that we now know that these diseases are largely preventable. The Surgeon General of the USA stated in 1987 that "......70% of diseases in the USA are diet related." This is an important admission and one that applies to all Westernised societies. If we accept this premise, it is sensible to consider the addition of essential nutrients to the diet, in the form of supplements. Vitamins, minerals, essential fatty acids, amino acids, fibres, bacteria, enzymes and herbs may all be added to the diet to help enhance the digestive processes, improve absorption and provide adequate levels of nutrients to help protect us against stress and pollution. The effects of these nutrients are described in the next chapter.

CHAPTER FOUR

YOUR PERSONAL CLEANSING PROGRAMME

W e wash our bodies, clean our teeth, wash our hair, and blow our noses, but how often do we clean out our body's digestive and waste disposal system? For thousands of years man has understood the importance of a clean GI tract. For example, yogis in the Himalayas swallow a length of cloth and pass it out some time later, which helps them to clean out their insides. This is done after fasting and is followed by a cleansing diet of whole cooked rice and clarified butter to clean out any bits that may have been left behind.

INTERNAL CLEANSING

It is even more important for us to keep our GI tract clean, considering the type of foods that we eat and our everyday exposure to a toxic environment. The typical Western diet is high in refined carbohydrates, low in fibre, high in fat and high in mucus forming dairy products, grains, fish and meat products. This is the perfect recipe for clogging up the tiny gaps between the villi of the small intestine.

We are all subject to this clogging up and constipation, and would benefit from a good clean out. Fortunately there are other methods available for cleaning out the digestive system which fit better with a Western lifestyle, as most of us do not have the yogis experience or time. The two most popular are colonic irrigation and herb and fibre internal cleansing.

Colonic Irrigation

Essentially, this is an extensive enema. Warm water is passed very gently and carefully, by a qualified practitioner, up into the colon from the anus. The warm water softens the impacted waste matter on the inside surface of the colon and gradually it comes away. Six such enemas during a six week course pulls away much of the impacted material. As most of the contents of the bowel are purged during this exercise, it is important to have an implant of beneficial bacteria to repopulate the colon.

Colon Cleansing

This method incorporates the use of water, absorbent fibres, beneficial bacteria and herbs especially selected for their anti-inflammatory, cleansing and healing properties. When this combination of nutrients is taken for prolonged periods of between two and four months, it has a similar effect to colonic irrigation. Some say it is preferable as it is less invasive, easier to administer and also cleans out the small intestine where absorptive surfaces can also get clogged up. The inclusion of beneficial bacteria, especially the human strains, helps to repopulate the colon with the bacteria that we need to aid digestion and absorption, and to fight off any invading micro-organisms that try to set up home in our colon.

Fibre and Fitness

There are many advantages in having the correct amount of fibre in the GI tract. Bulk promotes good muscle tone and fast transit time. Toxic chemicals are absorbed and carried out of the system. Fibre reduces the speed at which nutrients are released into the bloodstream during digestion so blood nutrient levels become more balanced. This results in a reduction in the quantity of food eaten and better satisfaction for longer, so that snacks are less frequently required.

Low fibre diets allow for the quick release of sugars into the blood stream and the pancreas may over react and release large amounts of insulin into the blood. Insulin clears sugar from the blood into the cells ,where energy is made, But if the pancreas secretes too much, then blood sugar levels may drop too low. This is why symptoms of low blood sugar often occur after eating food. This condition, termed *glucose intolerance* , is known to be the state that immediately preceeds many cases of adult onset diabetes.

Glucose Intolerance

It is becoming increasingly recognised that glucose intolerance can underlie many disease states, including premenstrual syndrome, some forms of schizophrenia, candidiasis, depression, anxiety, behaviour disturbances, allergies, severe mood swings and almost any condition where our thoughts or emotions are affected. This is because the brain and central nervous system rely almost entirely on blood glucose for energy and if blood glucose levels drop the brain becomes undernourished and unable to function properly.

Much success has been achieved employing high fibre, high complex carbohydrate, low fat and adequate protein diets in the treatment of glucose intolerance. Even the more wholesome Western diets are still unable to provide optimum levels of fibre. Oat bran, pectin, psyllium husks, glucomannan, beet fibre and guar gum are all highly absorbant and non aggressive fibres and useful to supplement for improved digestive health and glucose tolerance. Contrary to popular opinion, wheat bran is a poor absorber, is aggressive to the digestive tissues and can bind to calcium and zinc making them unavailable for absorption.

Once the GI tract is clean and the bacterial colony is balanced, digestive fitness can be maintained by eating a diet high in raw vegetables, fruits, seeds, nuts, sprouted legumes and whole grains, and low in meat, fish, dairy produce and refined, processed foods. If care is also taken to reduce or eliminate tea, coffee, alcohol and sugar while maintaining a good basic exercise programme, then a yearly spring clean should be enough to maintain continuous digestive health and efficiency.

MAXIMISING DIGESTION

To get the best from your food and supplements you need to have efficient digestive processes. In the mouth food needs to be well chewed so that it is broken up into smaller and more manageable pieces. Good stomach acid levels are essential for all mineral absorption. Diets high in protein encourage high acid levels as long as there is adequate vitamin B6 and zinc. If there is not, then stomach acid levels drop, protein is improperly digested and minerals may not be released for absorption. Low stomach acid is common in modern man.

The Acid Test

If you suspect that you have low levels of stomach acid, betaine hydrochloride (an amino acid that readily gives up its acid portion) and pepsin as a supplement may be of help. This will encourage better protein digestion and mineral absorption so that you will soon be making better levels of acid yourself. This should lead to a gradual relief from symptoms. If you have high acid levels and try this then your symptoms will temporarily worsen and you should stop the treatment. Your problem may lie elsewhere.

Panic in the Pancreas

Modern eating habits place an enormous demand on the pancreas to produce digestive enzymes. With the added burden of stressors and vitamin and mineral deficiency, as we age it becomes increasingly difficult for the pancreas to supply the demand and it can become exhausted. This leads to a risk that, proteins, carbohydrates and fats will not be completely digested, however good your stomach acid.

Undigested fats will readily clog up the villi and coat other food particles, inhibiting further digestion. Peptides, from improperly digested protein, can be absorbed and provoke allergies as well as providing food for putrefactive bacteria. Undigested starches are good for promoting the bacteria we do not want.

Breaking the Cycle

A diet low in starches, protein and fat and high in complex carbohydrates from vegetables will help to reduce the load on the system and stop the vicious cycle. Vitamins and minerals in amounts greater than can be provided by diet are usually required to promote the manufacture of enzymes. All the B complex vitamins, zinc, magnesium, chromium, manganese and iron are needed. It may also be very helpful to supplement digestive enzymes such as lipase, amylase and protease to support a weakened pancreas while the more long term benefits of the above are established.

CONTROLLING CANDIDA ALBICANS

There is really only one way to control Candida Albicans - create the correct conditions in the digestive system so that bacterial balance is achieved, boost the immune system, and ensure that candida's favourite diet of sugar is kept to an absolute minimum.

For those who do not have a candida problem this can be achieved by eating as "fundamentally" as is enjoyable - avoiding stressors, supplementing vitamins and minerals to support a healthy immune system, and taking regular, but not excessive, exercise.

For those with a candida problem there are other important factors to consider if you wish to rid yourself of this unwelcome guest.

Sugar

This is the single most important factor to remove from the diet. Without sugar, yeasts cannot survive. For our purposes here, sugar encompasses:

Sucrose - this is refined sugar of any colour and from any source. It is found in many processed foods and some that might surprise you, including honey.

Lactose - Milk sugar found in all milk and products that contain milk.

Fructose - Fruit sugar, though better for you than sucrose, provides sugar for yeasts and so concentrated fruit juices should be avoided. Dried fruit is best soaked and then eaten infrequently. For the first month on an anti-candida diet all fruit should be avoided.

Refined Foods

When grains are refined, all the fibre and most of the essential nutrients are removed, leaving only the starch. This starch now behaves like sugar in the GI tract and provides food for yeasts. Refined grains include white flour and any of its products, white and green pasta, white rice and potato starch (cooked and peeled potato, instant mash).

Yeasty Foods

Fermented foods and foods containing yeasts should be avoided for the best anti-candida results. These include levened bread, soy sauce, alcoholic beverages (even though spirits are not fermented they encourage poor glucose tolerance) especially sweet wines and beers, vinegar, mushrooms, vitamins derived from yeast, pickles, ketchup, yeast extracts and live foods that may be old and contain moulds - nuts and seeds should be checked for freshness. Cheeses are not recommended.

Antibiotics

As the name suggests these are drugs that kill living things and they are most effective against bacteria. When they are prescribed for infections and acne, or eaten in meat and dairy products, they may well kill off invading organisms. However they also kill off our friendly bacteria and leave us open to invasion. Candida Albicans takes advantage of this.

Steroid Drugs

These include medicinal drugs like cortisone, as well as the contraceptive pill and the hormone replacement therapy used by post-menopausal women. These disturb the acidity of the GI tract and encourage the growth of yeasts.

Natural Remedies

Fortunately treating Candida Albicans is not just a matter of eliminating everything that you like to eat from your diet. There are some very potent anti-candida nutrients some of which have only recently been discovered while others are ancient natural remedies.

- Olive oil - contains oleic acid, a fat which stops the conversion of the yeast form of Candida Albicans into its damaging fungal form. One to two tablespoons daily as a salad dressing is enough.

- Garlic - the healing and cleansing properties of garlic have been known for thousands of years. It is a very effective anti-bacterial and anti-yeast substance. Supplements of concentrated, deodorised garlic are now available.

- Bacteria - our own gut bacteria are best, but if levels are reduced, the addition of acidophilus bacteria from yoghurt helps to repopulate the gut. Human strains of beneficial bacteria are much more efficient at re-establishing the correct balance. These are available as supplements.

- Caprylic- Acid a fatty acid found in coconut that has the ability to kill Candida Albicans. It is now used in preference to anti-fungal drugs by many practitioners.

- Biotin - this B vitamin has similar anti-yeast properties to olive oil. 300mcg three times daily is good.

Defeating the Beastly Yeast

In summary, then, the following guidelines will help you to instigate a diet and supplement regime for the control of Candida Albicans:

1. Avoid all sugar - check for hidden sugar added to foods.

2. For the first month avoid fruit and fruit juices. These may be reintroduced if symptoms have improved. Fruit juice should always be diluted by half with water.

3. Avoid refined and processed foods and foods produced by or made from yeasts.

4. Eat plenty of natural, raw foods and keep animal products to a minimum. Natural live yoghurt can be introduced once symptoms have improved.

5. A colon cleanse is optional and greatly enhances the effects of all these other factors.

6. Take supplements of concentrated garlic, caprylic acid, beneficial bacteria and immune boosting nutrients. Health+Plus Ltd make a special supplement pack called CANTROL which provides these factors. Their address is on page 47.

7. Don't consume alcohol regularly. Have a couple of glasses of quality dry white wine as an occasional treat.

8. Follow these guidelines for at least three months. It may take as long as a year to clear the system of Candida Albicans. If in any doubt, contact a qualified nutrition consultant.

THE THIRTY DAY SPRING CLEAN

Week by week you can revitalise your diet, improve digestion and absorption and begin the cleansing process. You'll notice that your ability to taste foods will improve. You'll lose the urge to eat devitalised foods and experience choosing foods with much more consciousness, weighing up their potential health benefits and hazards. Once completed this diet can positively change your eating habits for the rest of your life.

This is your personal cleansing programme and is designed to be enjoyable as well as health promoting. Experience has shown that gradual changes are the most permanent, so if the pace of the diet is too fast for your liking then please adjust according to your needs. Get from it what you can. You can always adhere more closely to it when you repeat it next year. Each component of this programme is health promoting in itself. When they are all added together then they have even greater potency.

WEEK 1

INCREASE

Fresh fruit. Three pieces per day. These may take the form of breakfast, lunch or snacks. Apples and bananas are high in pectin.

Fresh vegetables. These are best lightly steamed or made into soups and salads.

Fresh fish. Herring, mackerel, sardine, tuna, haddock, cod and other deep sea fish are the least polluted and most nutritious. Shellfish and flat fish live in polluted coastal waters.

Whole grains (try some of the varieties available other than wheat) and their products.

Nuts and seeds. These can be added to salads or made up with wholegrains to make muesli.

Filtered or spring water.

Natural, live yoghurt. The highest levels of beneficial bacteria are found in brands that state 'live' on the pot.

Cold pressed olive and seed oils for salad dressings and dips.

43

DECREASE

Sugar and foods containing sugar.
Refined and devitalised foods.
Foods containing artificial additives.
Coffee, tea, alcohol, salt and dairy products. There are tasty fruit teas and coffee substitutes to discover.
Concentrated fruit juice. Dilute all natural juices with at least 50% filtered or spring water.
Red meats - beef, pork and lamb. Poultry is less fatty and free range is best.

SUPPLEMENTS

Take a good quality, strong multi-vitamin and multi mineral supplement daily with meals. It should contain at least the following.

B Complex	50mg
Vitamin C	1,000mg
Zinc	15mg
Calcium	150mg
Magnesium	100mg
Chromium	20mcg
Vitamin A	7,500iu
Vitamin E	100iu

Start an internal cleansing programme. This needs to include high strength beneficial bacteria. Various brands are available. The one I prefer is Health+Plus' ABSORB PLUS which provides herbs in a tablet, plus a combination of beet fibre, oat bran, guar gum, pectin and beneficial bacteria in a capsule. It is important to follow the instructions on the pack.

NOTE - changing to a more fibrous diet and starting a cleansing programme can cause some people to become temporarily constipated. Also mild elimination reactions may be felt such as headaches, irritability or tiredness. Please persevere. Turn to page 47 for books providing recipes compatible with this programme.

WEEK 2

Continue as for WEEK 1 and -

INCREASE

Raw foods. Legumes and grains can be sprouted by you or bought as sprouts. They need to be thoroughly cooked if unsprouted.
Water. Spring or filtered.
Garlic and onions, cooked and raw. They contain detoxifying nutrients.

DECREASE

All meats, fish and dairy produce.

AVOID

Coffee and tea.
All added sugar and foods containing it. Some fructose may be substituted
Foods containing artificial additives.

SUPPLEMENTS

Continue with internal cleanse as per instructions.
Continue with multivitamins and minerals.
Optional addition of digestive enzyme supplement, including amylase, lipase and protease enzymes.
Continue for the rest of the programme.

NOTE: Eat something raw, for example, a carrot before each cooked meal as this improves digestion.

WEEK 3

Continue as for WEEK 2 and -

INCREASE

Raw foods. These should now account for 40% of your diet.
Water. As much as you need to satisfy your thirst and for the fibre supplements.
Diluted fresh fruit juices to replace teas and coffees.

AVOID

Alcohol. Some dry white wine for treats is OK.
Meat, eggs and dairy produce bar live yoghurt and a little butter.

WEEK 4

Continue as for WEEK 3 and -

INCREASE

Live yoghurt.
Sprouted beans and seeds.
Exercise of your choice.

AVOID

Large meals. Eat until you feel satisfied and adjust the size of your meals accordingly.

NOTE: 60% of your diet should now be raw foods. The other 40% should be lightly steamed vegetables, live yoghurt, whole grains and their products. Soya milk is a good substitute for cow's milk. Tofu, soya bean curd, is a good source of protein. Your protein, essential fatty acid, energy, vitamin and mineral needs will be met if you follow this programme, providing you eat enough of the foods recommended.

WEEK 5 AND ONWARDS........

You can now begin to re-introduce foods that you have avoided but would like to eat once more. Please observe any changes that occur in well being or energy after these foods, as this may indicate an intolerance.

Please continue your internal cleansing programme for at least one more month - two would be preferable. If you continue to eat with the same degree of consciousness then you have every chance of maintaining your newly improved digestion and absorption.

FURTHER RECOMMENDED READING

Leslie and Susannah Keaton - *Raw Energy* - (Arrow Press) 1984. The authors present an interesting to read background on the benefits of eating raw food as well as a wealth of good recipe and food preparation ideas.

Doris Grant & Jean Joice - *Food Combining for Health* (Thorsons) 1984. This book explores the principles behind the work of Dr Hay and presents the evidence for the benefits of food combining. It contains plenty of interesting case histories and all the detail that you need if you want to follow Dr Hays recommendations closely, including lots of delicious recipes.

Pat Connolly - *The Candida Albicans Yeast Free Cook Book* (Keats). This is the only book of its kind available and essential if you wish to learn how to cook according to the anti-candida diet.

Patrick Holford - *The Metabolic Diet* (Ebury Press) 1987. This highly successful weight loss programme explains in simple terms the reason why we put weight on and what we can usefully do to redress the balance. It uses optimum nutrition and provides day to day recipes that are very compatible with the principles set out in this book.

Jennifer Meek - *How to Boost Your Immune System* (ION Press) 1988. This book explains how the immune system works and what to do to make yours healthy. It includes the Immune Power Diet .

USEFUL ADDRESSES

THE INSTITUTE FOR OPTIMUM NUTRITION (ION) offers courses and personal consultations with qualified nutritionists including the author, Christopher Scarfe. ION, 5 Jerdan Place, London, SW6 1BE. Tel. 01 385 7984.

HEALTH+PLUS LTD supply vitamin and mineral supplements by mail order. Health+Plus Ltd, Health+Plus House, 118 Station Road, Chinnor, OXON, OX9 4EZ. Tel. 0844 52098.

THE VEGETARIAN SOCIETY provide useful information of how to eat healthily as a vegetarian. 53 Marloes Road, London W8. Tel. 01 937 7739.

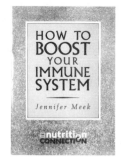
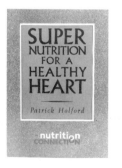
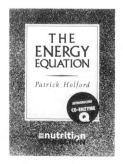